My Slow Cooker Everyday Desserts

A Collection of delicious Sweets and Desserts For Your Daily Meals

Donna Conway

© copyright 2021 – all rights reserved.

the content contained within this book may not be reproduced, duplicated or transmitted without direct written permission from the author or the publisher.

under no circumstances will any blame or legal responsibility be held against the publisher, or author, for any damages, reparation, or monetary loss due to the information contained within this book. either directly or indirectly.

legal notice:

this book is copyright protected. this book is only for personal use. you cannot amend, distribute, sell, use, quote or paraphrase any part, or the content within this book, without the consent of the author or publisher.

disclaimer notice:

please note the information contained within this document is for educational and entertainment purposes only. all effort has been executed to present accurate, up to date, and reliable, complete information. no warranties of any kind are declared or implied. readers acknowledge that the author is not engaging in the rendering of legal, financial, medical or professional advice. the content within this book has been derived from various sources. please consult a licensed professional before attempting any techniques outlined in this book.

by reading this document, the reader agrees that under no circumstances is the author responsible for any losses, direct or indirect, which are incurred as a result of the use of information contained within this document, including, but not limited to, — errors, omissions, or inaccuracies.

Table of Contents

BLUEBERRY DUMPLING PIE 6
BROWNED BUTTER PUMPKIN CHEESECAKE 8
BUTTER LIME CAKE 10
BUTTERSCOTCH CAKE 12
CARAMEL APPLE CRISP 14
CARAMEL PEAR PUDDING CAKE 16
COCONUT CONDENSED MILK CUSTARD 18
CHERRY ALMOND DESSERT OATMEAL 20
MOLTEN LAVA CAKE 22
MAPLE CRÉME BRÛLÉE 24
LEMON PUDDING CAKE 26
CHAI-SPICED PEARS 28
CRANBERRY WALNUT BREAD PUDDING 30
ALMOND BANANA BREAD 32
MAPLE ROASTED PEAR CRUMBLE 34
SUGARY MANDARIN & ALMOND PUDDING 36
SUGARY PLUMS 38
CARDAMOM PLUM CREAM 39
VANILLA RHUBARB MIX 40
PEACHES AND WHISKEY SAUCE 41
COCONUT CHOCOLATE CREAM 42
MAPLE CHERRY & COCOA COMPOTE 43
DATES CASHEW CAKE 45
NUTMEG APPLES 47
APPLE VANILLA CAKE 49
PEACH CRACKERS COBBLER 51
MILKY BLUEBERRY & ALMOND CAKE 53

Pears & Orange Sauce	55
Sugary Almond Cookies	56
Zesty Strawberries Marmalade	58
Cherry Cola Cake	59
Amaretti Cheesecake	61
Apple Cinnamon Brioche Pudding	63
Banana Walnut Cake	65
Black Forest Cake	67
Secret Chocolate Chili	69
Caveman's Chili	71
5-Ingredient Chili	73
Blueberry Lemon Custard Cake	74
Keto Fudge	76
Dark Chocolate Cake	78
Pumpkin Pecan Spice Cake	80
Glazed Walnuts	82
Keto Granola	83
Maple Custard	85
Raspberry Cream Cheese Coffee Cake	87
Pumpkin Pie Bars	90
Lemon Custard	92
Apple Brown	94
Baked Custard	96
Caramel Rum Fondue	98
Triple Chocolate Mess	99
Rice Pudding	101
Caramel Pie	103
Berry Cobbler	105
Minty Hot Fudge Sundae Cake	107

Blueberry Dumpling Pie

Preparation time: 15 minutes

Cooking time: 5 hours

Servings: 4 people

Ingredients:

- ¼ cup light brown sugar
- ½ cup butter, chilled and cubed
- ½ teaspoon salt
- 1 ½ cups all-purpose flour
- 1 ½ pound fresh blueberries
- 1 tablespoon lemon zest
- 1 teaspoon baking powder
- 2 tablespoons cornstarch
- 2 tablespoons white sugar
- 2/3 cup buttermilk, chilled

Directions:

1. Combine the blueberries, cornstarch, brown sugar, and lemon zest in the slow cooker. For the dumpling topping, combine the flour, salt, baking powder, sugar, and butter in a container and mix until sandy.
2. Mix in the buttermilk and stir to mix. Drop a spoonful of batter over the blueberries, switch your slow cooker to a low setting, and cook for about 5 hours. Allow the dessert to cool before you serve.

Nutrition:

Calories: 320

Carbs: 41g

Fat: 16g

Protein: 3g

Browned Butter Pumpkin Cheesecake

Preparation time: 15 minutes

Cooking time: 6 hours

Servings: 4 people

Ingredients:

Crust:

- ½ cup butter
- 1 ¼ cups crushed graham crackers

Filling:

- ¼ cup butter
- ½ cup light brown sugar
- ½ teaspoon cardamom powder
- 1 cup pumpkin puree
- 1 pinch salt
- 1 teaspoon cinnamon powder
- 1 teaspoon ground ginger

- 24 oz. cream cheese
- 4 eggs

Directions:

1. For the crust, start by browning the butter. Put the butter in a saucepan and cook for a few minutes until it starts to look golden. Let cool slightly.
2. Combine the browned butter with crushed crackers, then move the mixture in your slow cooker and press it well on the bottom of the pot.
3. For the filling, brown ¼ cup butter as described above, mix in the pumpkin puree, cream cheese, eggs, sugar, salt, cinnamon, ginger, and cardamom.
4. Pour the mixture over the crust, switch your slow cooker to low, and cook for about 6 hours. Let the cheesecake cool down before you slice and serve.

Nutrition: Calories: 142 Carbs: 23g Fat: 2g Protein: 11g

Butter Lime Cake

Preparation time: 15 minutes

Cooking time: 2 hours

Servings: 4 people

Ingredients:

- ¼ teaspoon salt
- 1 ¼ cups white sugar
- 1 ½ cups all-purpose flour
- 1 cup butter, softened
- 1 cup buttermilk
- 1 lime, zested and juiced
- 1 teaspoon baking powder
- 1 teaspoon vanilla extract
- 3 eggs

Directions:

1. Combine the butter and sugar in a container until creamy, for about 2 minutes. Put in the eggs, one by

one, then mix in the vanilla, buttermilk, lime zest, and lime juice.

2. Fold in the rest of the ingredients, then pour the batter into a greased slow cooker. Secure the lid, switch the slow cooker to high, and cook for about 2 hours. Let the cake cool in the pot before you serve.

Nutrition:

Calories: 286

Carbs: 63g

Fat: 2g

Protein: 5g

Butterscotch Cake

Preparation time: 15 minutes

Cooking time: 4 hours

Servings: 4 people

Ingredients:

- ½ cup butter softened
- ½ cup white sugar
- ½ cup whole milk
- ½ teaspoon salt
- 1 ½ cups all-purpose flour
- 1 cup butterscotch chocolate chips, melted
- 1 cup hot water
- 1 teaspoon baking powder

Directions:

1. Combine the butter and sugar in a container until creamy, at least 5 minutes. Put in the melted

butterscotch chips, then mix in the milk and hot water.

2. Fold in the flour, salt, and baking powder, then pour the batter into your slow cooker—Bake for about 4 hours on low. Let cool completely before you serve.

Nutrition:

Calories: 211

Carbs: 42g

Fat: 4g

Protein: 2g

Caramel Apple Crisp

Preparation time: 15 minutes

Cooking time: 6 hours

Servings: 4 people

Ingredients:

- ¼ cup butter, chilled
- ½ cup caramel sauce
- ½ cup rolled oats
- ½ teaspoon cinnamon powder
- 1 cup all-purpose flour
- 1 pinch salt
- 1 tablespoon cornstarch
- 6 Granny Smith apples, peeled, cored, and sliced

Directions:

1. Combine the apples, caramel sauce, cinnamon, and cornstarch in the slow cooker. For the topping,

combine the flour, oats, butter, and salt in a container until grainy.

2. Spread the topping over the apples, switch your slow cooker to a low setting and cook for about six hours. Allow the crisp to cool in the pot before you serve.

Nutrition:

Calories: 160

Carbs: 31g

Fat: 1g

Protein: 5g

Caramel Pear Pudding Cake

Preparation time: 15 minutes

Cooking time: 4 hours

Servings: 4 people

Ingredients:

- ¼ cup butter, melted
- ¼ cup whole milk
- ¼ teaspoon salt
- ½ cup of sugar
- ½ teaspoon cinnamon powder
- ¾ cup caramel sauce
- 1 teaspoon baking powder
- 2/3 cup all-purpose flour
- 4 ripe pears, cored and sliced

Directions:

1. Mix the flour, baking powder, sugar, salt, plus cinnamon in a container. Put in the butter and milk and stir to mix.
2. Put the pears in your slow cooker and top with the batter. Drizzle the batter with caramel sauce, switch your slow cooker to low, and cook for about 4 hours. Let the cake cool before you serve.

Nutrition:

Calories: 223

Carbs: 42g

Fat: 6g

Protein: 2g

Coconut Condensed Milk Custard

Preparation time: 15 minutes

Cooking time: 5 hours

Servings: 4 people

Ingredients:

- 1 ¼ cups sweetened condensed milk
- 1 can (15 oz.) coconut milk
- 1 cup evaporated milk
- 1 tablespoon vanilla extract
- 1 teaspoon lime zest
- 6 eggs

Directions:

1. Combine the eggs, coconut milk, condensed milk, vanilla, lime zest, and evaporated milk in a container. Pour the mixture in the slow.

2. Secure the lid, switch your slow cooker to low, and cook for about 5 hours. Let cool before you serve.

Nutrition:

Calories: 154

Carbs: 26g

Fat: 5g

Protein: 0g

Cherry Almond Dessert Oatmeal

Preparation time: 15 minutes

Cooking time: 7 hours

Servings: 4 people

Ingredients:

- 2 cups vanilla almond milk
- 1 ½ cups water
- 1 cup steel-cut oats
- ¾ cup dried tart cherries
- ½ cup unsweetened organic applesauce
- 1 tablespoon ground flax seed
- ½ teaspoon pure almond extract
- Pinch of salt
- A drizzle of organic honey

Directions:

1. Grease your slow cooker with a coconut-oil based spray. Add everything to the cooker except honey and cover. Cook on low for 7 hours. When time is up, divide into bowls, drizzle each with honey, and serve!

Nutrition:

Calories: 186

Protein: 3 g

Carbs: 32 g

Fat: 3 g

Molten Lava Cake

Preparation time: 15 minutes

Cooking time: 2 hours

Servings: 4 people

Ingredients:

Cake:

- 2 cups oat flour
- 1 ½ cups organic coconut sugar
- 1 cup unsweetened coconut milk
- 6 tablespoons organic cocoa powder
- 4 tablespoons grass-fed melted butter
- 1 tablespoon baking powder
- 2 teaspoons vanilla
- 1 teaspoon salt

Sauce:

- 2 cups boiling water
- ¾ cup of organic coconut sugar

- ½ cup organic cocoa powder
- ¼ cup of organic honey

Directions:

1. Grease a slow cooker with a coconut-oil based cooker. In a bowl, mix flour, cocoa, sugar, salt, and baking powder.
2. Add in melted butter, vanilla, and coconut milk until smooth. Pour into the slow cooker. In another bowl, looking to the sauce list, mix cocoa powder and sugar. Sprinkle over cake batter. In a third bowl, mix honey and boiling water.
3. Pour over the cake without mixing, and cover the lid. Cook on high for 1 ½-2 hour. You can tell the cake is done when it's puffed up and firm on top, with the sauce having sunk to the bottom. Serve warm!

Nutrition: Calories: 317 Protein: 5 g Carbs: 65 g Fat: 7 g

Maple Créme Brûlée

Preparation time: 15 minutes

Cooking time: 2 hours & 30 minutes

Servings: 3 people

Ingredients:

Créme:

- Boiling water
- 1 1/3 cups heavy whipping cream
- 3 egg yolks
- ½ cup of coconut sugar
- ½ teaspoon pure organic maple extract
- ¼ teaspoon cinnamon

Topping:

- 3 teaspoons coconut sugar

Directions:

1. In a saucepan, heat cream until the sides begin to bubble on the sides gently. While that is getting hot, whisk eggs, yolks, sugar, and cinnamon together.
2. When the cream is forming bubbles on the side, then remove it from heat. Stir a little of this hot cream into the yolks.
3. Pour yolks into the pan and constantly whisk to integrate, then put the maple. Move créme into 6-oz. ramekins.
4. Put in your slow cooker and pour in one inch's worth of boiling water. Cook on high for 2 hours and 30 minutes hours until the ramekins jiggle, but the center is set.
5. Cool for 10 minutes outside of the cooker before wrapping in saran wrap and refrigerating for 4 hours.
6. When you're ready to eat, add 1 teaspoon of sugar per ramekin on top, and Brulee with a torch. Enjoy!

Nutrition: Calories: 578 Protein: 5g Carbs: 44g Fat: 44g

Lemon Pudding Cake

Preparation time: 15 minutes

Cooking time: 2 hours

Servings: 4 people

Ingredients:

- 2/3 cup plain Greek yogurt
- 2 egg yolks
- 2 egg whites
- ½ cup of coconut sugar
- ¼ cup flour
- 1 lemon's worth of juice and zest
- ¼ teaspoon salt
- Water

Directions:

1. Grease four 6-ounce ramekins. In a bowl, whisk flour, salt, and sugar. In another bowl, mix egg yolks, yogurt, lemon juice, and lemon zest.
2. When smooth, add dry ingredients into wet until just mixed. In another bowl, beat the egg whites until you get stiff peaks.
3. Fold whites into the batter. Divide batter into the ramekins and set in your slow cooker. Put in just enough water to reach the halfway mark.
4. Close lid and cook on low for 2 hours. Cool for 10 minutes before serving!

Nutrition:

Calories: 216

Protein: 6g

Carbs: 35g

Fat: 6g

Chai-Spiced Pears

Preparation time: 15 minutes

Cooking time: 3-4 hours

Servings: 4 people

Ingredients:

- 4 pears
- 2 cups fresh orange juice
- 5 whole cardamom pods
- ¼ cup pure maple syrup
- 1-inch piece of sliced peeled ginger
- 1 halved cinnamon stick

Directions:

1. Peel pears and cut off the bottom so it stands up in the slow cooker. Carefully remove the cores without destroying the fruit.

2. Put pears in the slow cooker, standing up. Add the rest of the ingredients, spooning some juice over the top of the pears.
3. Cook on low for 3-4 hours, basting again with liquid every hour. When the pears are soft, they're done!

Nutrition:

Calories: 253

Protein: 2g

Carbs: 61g

Fat: 1g

Cranberry Walnut Bread Pudding

Preparation time: 15 minutes

Cooking time: 4 hours

Servings: 4 people

Ingredients:

- 5 cups cubed whole-wheat (or whole-grain) bread
- 2 ½ cups whole organic milk
- 3 beaten organic eggs
- ½ cup unsweetened dried cranberries
- ½ cup chopped walnuts
- ½ cup pure maple syrup
- ½ cup grass-fed butter
- 1 teaspoon pure vanilla extract
- Dash of cinnamon

Directions:

1. In a bowl, whisk milk, eggs, syrup, cinnamon, and vanilla together. Add bread and press it down so it's submerged. Soak for 10 minutes.
2. In the meantime, grease your slow cooker with a coconut-oil based spray. When 10 minutes have passed, add nuts and cranberries to the pudding.
3. Pour into the slow cooker—Cook for 4 hours on low.
4. Add butter to a saucepan. Cook on medium, stirring every once and a while, to get brown butter. The butter will become aromatic, like a caramel, and get an amber color. Serve.

Nutrition:

Calories: 488

Protein: 8g

Carbs: 35g

Fat: 26g

Almond Banana Bread

Preparation time: 15 minutes

Cooking time: 4 hours

Servings: 4 people

Ingredients:

- 3 mashed bananas
- 2 cups whole-wheat flour
- 2 organic eggs
- 1 cup of organic coconut sugar
- ¾ cup sliced almonds
- ½ cup grass-fed softened butter
- 1 teaspoon baking powder
- 1 teaspoon pure almond extract
- ½ teaspoon baking soda
- ½ teaspoon salt
- ¼ teaspoon cinnamon
- 1/8 teaspoon nutmeg

Directions:

1. Grease your slow cooker with a coconut-oil based spray. In a large bowl, mix sugar, eggs, butter, and almond extract.
2. Add in baking soda, baking powder, salt, nutmeg, and cinnamon. Stir in flour. Stir in your mashed bananas and almonds.
3. Move batter to your slow cooker and cover with 3 paper towels—Cook for 4 hours on low.
4. When time is up, carefully turning the slow cooker pot upside down on a plate to remove the bread. Serve at room temperature or cold!

Nutrition:

Calories: 570

Protein: 11g

Carbs: 85g

Fat: 23g

Maple Roasted Pear Crumble

Preparation time: 15 minutes

Cooking time: 4 hours & 30 minutes

Servings: 4 people

Ingredients:

- 6 firm pears, cut in half
- ½ cup of water
- ¼ cup pure maple syrup
- 1 teaspoon pure vanilla extract
- 1 teaspoon cinnamon
- ½ teaspoon ginger
- ¼ teaspoon nutmeg

Crumble:

- 2/3 cups rolled oats
- 2 tablespoons organic coconut sugar
- 1 tablespoon pure maple syrup
- 1 tablespoon coconut oil

Directions:

1. Put all the fixings in the first list in the slow cooker. Cook on high within 1 hour, and then switch to low for 4 hours. When done, put pears and some cooking liquid in an 8x8 baking dish.
2. For the crumble, pulse the ingredients in the second list in a food processor until oats are sticky. Sprinkle topping on pears and bake in a 350-degree oven for 30 minutes. Serve!

Nutrition:

Calories: 260

Protein: 2g

Carbs: 57g

Fat: 3g

Sugary Mandarin & Almond Pudding

Preparation time: 10 minutes

Cooking time: 2 hours and 30 minutes

Servings: 2 people

Ingredients:

- ½ mandarin, sliced
- Juice of 1 mandarin
- 1 tablespoon sugar
- 2 oz. butter, soft
- 1 egg
- ½ cup of sugar
- ½ cup flour
- ½ teaspoon baking powder
- ½ cup almonds, ground
- Cooking spray

Directions:

1. Grease your slow cooker with cooking spray, sprinkle half of the sugar on the bottom, and arrange mandarin slices.
2. In a bowl, mix butter with the rest of the sugar, egg, almonds, flour, baking powder, and the mandarin juice and whisk well
3. Spread this over mandarin slices, cover, cook on high for 2 hours and 30 minutes, transfer to a platter, and serve cold. Enjoy!

Nutrition:

Calories: 200

Fat: 4g

Carbs: 8g

Protein: 6g

Sugary Plums

Preparation time: 10 minutes

Cooking time: 3 hours

Servings: 2 people

Ingredients:

- 6 plums, halved and pitted
- ½ cup of sugar
- 1 teaspoon cinnamon, ground
- ¼ cup of water
- 1 tablespoon cornstarch

Directions:

1. Put plums in your slow cooker, add sugar, cinnamon, water, and cornstarch, stir, cover, and cook on low for 3 hours. Serve as a dessert.

Nutrition: Calories: 180 Fat: 2g Carbs: 8g Protein: 8g

Cardamom Plum Cream

Preparation time: 10 minutes

Cooking time: 7 hours

Servings: 2 people

Ingredients:

- 1 and ½ pounds plums, pitted and halved
- ½ cup of water
- ¼ teaspoon cinnamon, ground
- ¼ teaspoon cardamom, ground
- ¼ cup of sugar

Directions:

1. Put plums and water in your slow cooker, cover, and cook on low for 1 hour. Add cinnamon, sugar, and cardamom, stir, cover, cook on low for 6 hours more, divide into jars and serve. Enjoy!

Nutrition: Calories: 280 Fat: 2g Carbs: 10g Protein: 6g

Vanilla Rhubarb Mix

Preparation time: 10 minutes

Cooking time: 6 hours

Servings: 4 people

Ingredients:

- 2 cups rhubarb, chopped
- 1 tablespoon butter, melted
- ¼ cup of water
- ½ cup of sugar
- ½ teaspoon vanilla extract

Directions:

1. Put rhubarb in your slow cooker, add water and sugar, stir gently, cover, and cook on low for 6 hours. Add butter and vanilla, stir and keep in the fridge until it's cold. Enjoy!

Nutrition: Calories: 200 Fat: 2g Carbs: 6g Protein: 1g

Peaches and Whiskey Sauce

Preparation time: 10 minutes

Cooking time: 2 hours

Servings: 2 people

Ingredients:

- ½ cup brown sugar
- 1 and ½ cups peaches, pitted and cut into wedges
- 3 tablespoons whiskey
- ½ cup white sugar
- 1 teaspoon lemon zest, grated

Directions:

1. In your slow cooker, mix peaches with brown and white sugar, whiskey, and lemon zest, stir, cover, and cook on high for 2 hours. Divide into bowls and serve warm.

Nutrition: Calories: 200 Fat: 4g Carbs: 9g Protein: 4g

Coconut Chocolate Cream

Preparation time: 10 minutes

Cooking time: 1 hour

Servings: 2 people

Ingredients:

- 2 oz. coconut cream
- 2 oz. dark chocolate, cut into chunks
- ½ teaspoon sugar

Directions:

1. In a bowl, mix coconut cream with chocolate and sugar, whisk well, pour into your slow cooker, cover, cook on high for 1 hour, divide into bowls and serve cold. Enjoy!

Nutrition: Calories: 242 Fat: 12g Carbs: 9g Protein: 4g

Maple Cherry & Cocoa Compote

Preparation time: 10 minutes

Cooking time: 2 hours

Servings: 2 people

Ingredients:

- ¼ cup of cocoa powder
- ½ cup red cherry juice
- 2 tablespoons maple syrup
- ½ pound cherries pitted and halved
- 1 tablespoon sugar
- 1 cups of water

Directions:

1. In your slow cooker, mix cocoa with cherry juice, maple syrup, cherries, water, and sugar, stir, cover, cook on high for 2 hours, divide into bowls and serve cold. Enjoy!

Nutrition:

Calories: 200

Fat: 1g

Carbs: 5g

Protein: 2g

Dates Cashew Cake

Preparation time: 10 minutes

Cooking time: 2 hours

Servings: 2 people

Ingredients:

For the base:

- ¼ cup dates pitted
- ½ tablespoon water
- ¼ teaspoon vanilla
- ¼ cup almonds

For the cake:

- 1 and ½ cups cashews, soaked for 8 hours
- ½ cup blueberries
- ½ cup maple syrup
- ½ tablespoon vegetable oil

Directions:

1. In your food processor, mix dates with water, vanilla, and almonds, pulse well, transfer it to a working surface, flatten and arrange it on the bottom of your slow cooker.
2. In your blender, mix maple syrup with coconut oil, cashews, and blueberries, blend well, spread over crust, cover, and cook on high for 2 hours. Leave the cake to cool down, slice, and serve.

Nutrition:

Calories: 200

Fat: 3g

Carbs: 12g

Protein: 3g

Nutmeg Apples

Preparation time: 10 minutes

Cooking time: 1 hour

Servings: 2 people

Ingredients:

- ½ teaspoon cinnamon powder
- 3 oz. apples, cored and chopped
- 1 egg, whisked
- ¼ cup whipping cream
- 1 tablespoon sugar
- ½ teaspoon nutmeg, ground
- 1 teaspoon vanilla extract
- 2 tablespoons pecans, chopped

Directions:

1. In your slow cooker, mix cream, vanilla, nutmeg, sugar, apples, egg, and cinnamon, stir, cover, cook on

high for 1 hour, divide into bowls, sprinkle pecans on top, and serve cold. Enjoy!

Nutrition:

Calories: 260

Fat: 3g

Carbs: 14g

Protein: 3g

Apple Vanilla Cake

Preparation time: 10 minutes

Cooking time: 2 hours and 30 minutes

Servings: 2 people

Ingredients:

- 1 and ½ cups apples, cored and cubed
- 1 and ½ tablespoons sugar
- 1 tablespoon vanilla extract
- 1 egg
- ½ tablespoon apple pie spice
- 1 cup white flour
- ½ tablespoon baking powder
- ½ tablespoon butter, melted

Directions:

1. In a bowl, mix eggs with butter, pie spice, vanilla, apples, and sugar and stir using your mixer. In

another bowl, mix baking powder with flour, stir, add to apple mix, stir again well, transfer to your slow cooker, cover, cook on high for 2 hours and 30 minutes, leave cake aside to cool down, slice, and serve.

Nutrition:

Calories: 200

Fat: 2g

Carbs: 5g

Protein: 4g

Peach Crackers Cobbler

Preparation time: 10 minutes

Cooking time: 4 hours

Servings: 2 people

Ingredients:

- 2 cups peaches, peeled and sliced
- 3 tablespoons sugar
- ½ teaspoon cinnamon powder
- 1 cup sweet crackers, crushed
- ¼ teaspoon nutmeg, ground
- ¼ cup milk
- 1 teaspoon vanilla extract
- Cooking spray

Directions:

1. In a bowl, mix peaches with half of the sugar and cinnamon and stir. In another bowl, combine

crackers with the rest of the sugar, nutmeg, almond milk, and vanilla extract and stir.
2. Oiled your slow cooker with cooking spray, spread peaches on the bottom, add crackers mix, spread, cover, and cook on low for 4 hours. Divide cobbler between plates and serve.

Nutrition:

Calories: 212

Fat: 4g

Carbs: 7g

Protein: 3g

Milky Blueberry & Almond Cake

Preparation time: 10 minutes

Cooking time: 1 hour

Servings: 2 people

Ingredients:

- ¼ cup flour
- ¼ teaspoon baking powder
- ¼ teaspoon sugar
- ¼ cup blueberries
- ½ cup milk
- 1 teaspoon olive oil
- ½ teaspoon lemon zest, grated
- ¼ teaspoon vanilla extract
- ¼ teaspoon lemon extract
- Cooking spray

Directions:

1. In a bowl, mix flour with baking powder and sugar and stir. Add blueberries, milk, oil, lemon zest, vanilla extract, and lemon extract and whisk well.
2. Spray your slow cooker with cooking spray, line it with parchment paper, pour cake batter, cover pot, and cook on high for 1 hour. Leave the cake to cool down, slice, and serve.

Nutrition:

Calories: 200

Fat: 4g

Carbs: 10g

Protein: 4g

Pears & Orange Sauce

Preparation time: 10 minutes

Cooking time: 4 hours

Servings: 2 people

Ingredients:

- 2 pears, peeled and cored
- 1 cup of orange juice
- 2 tablespoons maple syrup
- 1 teaspoon cinnamon powder
- ½ tablespoon ginger, grated

Directions:

1. In your slow cooker, mix pears with orange juice, maple syrup, cinnamon, ginger, cover, and cook on low for 4 hours. Divide pears and sauce between plates and serve warm.

Nutrition: Calories: 250 Fat: 1g Carbs: 12g Protein: 4g

Sugary Almond Cookies

Preparation time: 10 minutes

Cooking time: 2 hours and 30 minutes

Servings: 2 people

Ingredients:

- 1 tablespoon vegetable oil
- 2 eggs
- ¼ cup of sugar
- ¼ teaspoon vanilla extract
- ¼ teaspoon baking powder
- 1 cup flour
- ¼ cup almonds, chopped

Directions:

1. In a bowl, mix oil with sugar, vanilla extract, and eggs and whisk. Add baking powder, almond meal, and almonds and stir well.

2. Line your slow cooker with parchment paper, spread cookie mix on the bottom of the pot, cover, cook on low for 2 hours and 30 minutes, leave aside to cool down, cut into medium pieces and serve.

Nutrition:

Calories: 220

Fat: 2g

Carbs: 6g

Protein: 6g

Zesty Strawberries Marmalade

Preparation time: 10 minutes

Cooking time: 4 hours

Servings: 2 people

Ingredients:

- 5 oz. strawberries, chopped
- ¼ pound sugar
- Zest of ½ lemon, grated
- 1-ounce raisins
- 1 1/2 oz. water

Directions:

1. In your slow cooker, mix strawberries with sugar, lemon zest, raisins, water, stir, cover, and cook on high for 4 hours. Divide into small jars and serve cold.

Nutrition: Calories: 250 Fat: 3g Carbs: 6g Protein: 1g

Cherry Cola Cake

Preparation time: 15 minutes

Cooking time: 4 hours

Servings: 4 people

Ingredients:

- ¼ cup of cocoa powder
- ¼ cup light brown sugar
- ¼ teaspoon salt
- ½ cup butter, melted
- ½ cup whole milk
- ½ teaspoon baking powder
- ½ teaspoon baking soda
- 1 ½ cups all-purpose flour
- 1 cup cola
- 1 teaspoon vanilla extract
- 2 cups cherries, pitted

Directions:

1. Combine the cola, sugar, butter, vanilla, and milk in a container. Put in the flour, cocoa powder, salt, baking powder, and baking soda and stir to mix.
2. Fold in the cherries. Spoon the batter in your slow cooker, switch your slow cooker to low, and cook for about 4 hours. Let the cake cool in the pot before you slice and serve.

Nutrition:

Calories: 440

Carbs: 62g

Fat: 21g

Protein: 3g

Amaretti Cheesecake

Preparation time: 15 minutes

Cooking time: 6 hours

Servings: 4 people

Ingredients:

Crust:

- ¼ cup butter, melted
- 6 oz. Amaretti cookies, crushed

Filling:

- ½ cup sour cream
- ½ cup white sugar
- 1 tablespoon Amaretto liqueur
- 1 tablespoon vanilla extract
- 24 oz. cream cheese
- 4 eggs

Directions:

1. Combine the crushed cookies with butter, then move the mixture to your slow cooker and press it well on the bottom of the pot.
2. For the filling, combine the cream cheese, sour cream, eggs, sugar, vanilla, and liqueur and stir to mix.
3. Pour the filling over the crust and cook for about six hours on low settings. Let the cheesecake cool before you slice and serve.

Nutrition:

Calories: 232

Carbs: 32g

Fat: 24g

Protein: 11g

Apple Cinnamon Brioche Pudding

Preparation time: 15 minutes

Cooking time: 6 hours

Servings: 4 people

Ingredients:

- ½ teaspoon ground ginger
- 1 cup evaporated milk
- 1 cup sweetened condensed milk
- 1 cup whole milk
- 1 teaspoon cinnamon powder
- 1 teaspoon vanilla extract
- 16 oz. brioche bread, cubed
- 2 tablespoons white sugar
- 4 eggs
- 4 Granny Smith apples, peeled and cubed

Directions:

1. Combine the brioche bread, apples, cinnamon, ginger, and sugar in your slow cooker. Mix the 3 types of milk in a container. Put in the eggs and vanilla and mix thoroughly.
2. Pour this mix over the bread, then cover the pot and cook for about 6 hours on low settings. The pudding tastes best when slightly warm.

Nutrition:

Calories: 176

Carbs: 22g

Fat: 7g

Protein: 6g

Banana Walnut Cake

Preparation time: 15 minutes

Cooking time: 4 hours

Servings: 4 people

Ingredients:

- ¼ teaspoon salt
- ½ cup canola oil
- 1 ¼ cups all-purpose flour
- 1 cup chopped walnuts
- 1 cup white sugar
- 1 teaspoon baking powder
- 1 teaspoon vanilla extract
- 2 eggs
- 4 small ripe bananas, mashed

Directions:

1. Mix the sugar plus oil in a container for about two minutes, then add the eggs and continue mixing for a few minutes until fluffy.
2. Put in the vanilla and bananas, fold in the flour, baking powder and salt, and walnuts. Pour the batter into your slow cooker and bake for about 4 hours on low. Slice and serve.

Nutrition:

Calories: 120

Carbs: 24g

Fat: 3g

Protein: 1g

Black Forest Cake

Preparation time: 15 minutes

Cooking time: 4 hours

Servings: 4 people

Ingredients:

- ½ cup butter softened
- ½ cup of cocoa powder
- ½ teaspoon salt
- ¾ cup white sugar
- 1 cup all-purpose flour
- 1-pound pitted cherries
- 1 tablespoon cornstarch
- 1 teaspoon baking powder
- 1 teaspoon vanilla extract
- 2 tablespoons kirsch
- 3 eggs
- Whipped cream for serving

Directions:

1. Combine the cherries, kirsch, and cornstarch in the slow cooker. For the batter, combine the butter, sugar, and vanilla in a container until creamy.
2. Put in the eggs, fold in the rest of the ingredients, and not over-mix the batter. Spoon the batter over the cherries and cook for about 4 hours on low. Serve the cake chilled, with the topping of whipped cream.

Nutrition:

Calories: 295

Carbs: 30g

Fat: 18g

Protein: 4g

Secret Chocolate Chili

Preparation time: 15 minutes

Cooking time: 4 hours

Servings: 4 people

Ingredients:

- ½ onion
- 1 cup beef broth
- 1 cup black coffee
- 1 tbsp. chili powder
- 1 tbsp. cocoa powder
- 1 tbsp. soy sauce
- 1 tsp. cayenne pepper
- 1 tsp. cumin
- 10 drops liquid stevia
- 2 cans whole tomatoes
- 2-pounds ground beef
- 2 tbsp. butter

- 2 tbsp. Worcestershire sauce
- 2 tsp. garlic
- 2 tsp. paprika
- 6 slices of bacon
- 8-oz. kielbasa

Directions:

1. Puree both cans of tomatoes in a food processor and add to the slow cooker. Add spices and all liquid ingredients minus garlic and butter to sauce in the slow cooker.
2. Add stevia—brown beef in a pan. Drain and put to the side. Chop onion, then sauté it in a pan until softened.
3. Add bacon and kielbasa to the pan with the onion, cooking till bacon is crispy. Add sausage and bacon mixture along with garlic powder to slow cooker. Add beef to the slow cooker. Set to cook on high 4 hours.

Nutrition: Calories: 492 Carbs: 7g Fat: 25g Protein: 17g

Caveman's Chili

Preparation time: 15 minutes

Cooking time: 4 hours

Servings: 4 people

Ingredients:

- 1 ½ tsp cumin
- 1 cup beef broth
- 1 green pepper
- 1 onion
- 1 tsp. cayenne pepper
- 1 tsp. oregano
- 1 tsp. pepper
- 1 tsp. salt
- 1 tsp. Worcestershire sauce
- 1/3 cup tomato paste
- 2 ½ tbsp. chili powder
- 2-pounds stew meat

- 2 tbsp. olive oil
- 2 tbsp. soy sauce
- 2 tsp. fish sauce
- 2 tsp. minced garlic
- 2 tsp. paprika

Directions:

1. Chop up half of your meat into bite-sized pieces. Place the other half of your meat into your food processor, blending until ground.
2. Cut up onion and pepper into tiny pieces. Mix all your spices. Sauté beef in the pan along with ground beef.
3. Sauté veggies in meat grease until fragrant Add all ingredients into your slow cooker. Simmer on high for 2 ½ hours. Stir and simmer 20-30 more minutes.

Nutrition: Calories: 390 Carbs: 5g Fat: 16g Protein: 27g

5-Ingredient Chili

Preparation time: 15 minutes

Cooking time: 2-3 hours

Servings: 4 people

Ingredients:

- 15-oz. tomato sauce
- 2 diced onions
- Cumin and other spices to achieve desired taste, such as cilantro, garlic, salt, chili powder, etc.
- 3-4 cans diced tomatoes
- 3-4 pounds meat of choice (ground turkey, bison, sausage, venison, beef, etc.)

Directions:

1. Pour all ingredients into your slow cooker. Stir well to incorporate. Cook 2-3 hours on high or 5-6 hours on low.

Nutrition: Calories: 503 Carbs: 6g Fat: 41g Protein: 29g

Blueberry Lemon Custard Cake

Preparation time: 15 minutes

Cooking time: 3 hours

Servings: 12 slices

Ingredients:

- 6 eggs separated
- 1/2 cup Coconut Flour
- 2 tsp lemon zest
- 1/3 cup lemon juice
- 1 tsp lemon liquid stevia
- 1/2 cup Swerve sweetener
- 1/2 tsp salt
- 2 cups heavy cream
- 1/2 cup fresh blueberries

Directions:

1. Put the egg whites into your stand mixer and whip until stiff peaks form. Set aside. Mix the yolks and remaining fixings except for blueberries in another bowl.
2. Fold the egg whites into the batter until just combined. Oiled slow cooker and pour the mixture into it.
3. Sprinkle the blueberries over the batter—cover and cook on low within 3 hours or until a toothpick comes out clean.
4. Allow cooling with the cover off for 1 hour, then place in the refrigerator to chill for 2 hours or overnight. Serve cold with a little sugar-free whipped cream if desired.

Nutrition: Calories: 191 Fat: 17g Protein: 4g Carbs: 4g

Keto Fudge

Preparation time: 5 minutes

Cooking time: 2 hours

Servings: 4 people

Ingredients:

- 2 1/2 cups sugar-free chocolate chips
- 1/3 cup coconut milk
- 1 tsp. pure vanilla extract
- a dash of salt
- 2 teaspoons vanilla liquid stevia (optional)

Directions:

1. Mix coconut milk, chocolate chips, vanilla, stevia, plus salt in a slow cooker. Cover and cook on low within 2 hours.

2. Let it sit for 30 minutes to 1 hour. Stir well for 5 minutes until smooth.

3. Line a one-quart casserole dish with parchment paper and spread mixture. Chill 30 minutes or until firm. Serve and enjoy!

Nutrition:

Calories: 65

Fat: 5g

Protein: 1g

Carbs: 2g

Dark Chocolate Cake

Preparation time: 10 minutes

Cooking time: 3 hours

Servings: 10 slices

Slow cooker size: 6-quart

Ingredients:

- 1 cup plus 2 tbsp almond flour
- 1/2 cup Swerve Granular
- 1/2 cup cocoa powder
- 3 tbsp unflavored whey protein powder
- 1 1/2 tsp baking powder
- 1/4 tsp salt
- 6 tbsp butter melted
- 3 large eggs
- 2/3 cup unsweetened almond milk
- 3/4 tsp vanilla extract
- 1/3 cup sugar-free chocolate chips optional

Directions:

1. Oiled a 6-quart slow cooker. Mix almond flour, sweetener, cocoa powder, whey protein powder, baking powder, and salt in a medium bowl.
2. Mix in butter, eggs, almond milk plus vanilla extract, then mixes in chocolate chips, if using.
3. Put into the prepared slow cooker and cook on low within 2 to 2 1/2 hours. Turn the slow cooker off, let cold 20 to 30 minutes, and then cut into pieces and serve warm. Serve with lightly sweetened whipped cream.

Nutrition:

Calories: 205

Fat: 17g

Protein: 7.4g

Carbs: 8.4g

Pumpkin Pecan Spice Cake

Preparation time: 10 minutes

Cooking time: 3 hours

Servings: 4 people

Slow cooker size: 6-quart

Ingredients:

- 1 1/2 cups raw pecans
- 3/4 cup Swerve Sweetener
- 1/3 cup coconut flour
- 1/4 cup unflavored whey protein powder
- 2 tsp baking powder
- 1 1/2 tsp ground cinnamon
- 1 tsp ground ginger
- 1/4 tsp ground cloves
- 1/4 tsp salt
- 1 cup pumpkin puree
- 4 large eggs

- 1/4 cup butter melted
- 1 tsp vanilla extract

Directions:

1. Grease the ceramic liner of the 6-quart slow cooker or line with parchment paper.
2. Grind pecans using a food processor or high-powered blender. Transfer to a bowl and whisk in sweetener, coconut flour, whey protein powder, baking powder, cinnamon, ginger, cloves, and salt.
3. Stir in pumpkin puree, eggs, butter, and vanilla until well combined. Spread into the prepared slow cooker and set to low. Cook 2 1/2 to 3 hours, or until set and top is barely firm to the touch. Serve and enjoy!

Nutrition: Calories: 344 Fat: 30.4g Protein: 8.3g Carbs: 10g

Glazed Walnuts

Preparation time: 5 minutes

Cooking time: 2 hours

Servings: 4 people

Ingredients:

    16 oz. walnuts

    ½ cup butter

    ½ cup maple syrup

    1 tsp. vanilla extract

Directions:

1. Put the walnuts, butter, maple syrup, and vanilla extract into the slow cooker. Cook for 2 hours on low.
2. Stir every 25 minutes to be sure all the walnuts are covered and not burned. After the time is over, take the walnuts off and cool on parchment paper. Serve.

Nutrition: Calories: 205 Fat: 17g Protein: 7.4g Carbs: 8.4g

Keto Granola

Preparation time: 10 minutes

Cooking time: 2 hours

Servings: 4 people

Ingredients:

- 1/3 cup coconut oil
- 1 tsp vanilla extract
- 1 tsp vanilla stevia
- 1/2 cup almonds
- 1/2 cup walnuts
- 1/2 cup pecans
- 1/2 cup hazelnuts
- 1 cup sunflower seeds
- 1 cup pumpkin seeds
- 1 cup unsweetened shredded coconut
- 1/2 cup sweetener
- 1 tsp ground cinnamon

- 1 tsp salt

Directions:

1. Set your slow cooker to low, then put coconut oil, and allow it to melt. Once melted, add vanilla extract and stevia. Stir well before adding nuts, seeds, and coconut.
2. Stir the granola mixture well to make sure all is coated. Whisk the sweetener, cinnamon, and salt together, then sprinkle over the nut and seed mixture.
3. Cover and cook on low within 2 hours or until you can smell them and they appear browned and toasted. Stir every 30 minutes.
4. Pour and spread out onto a baking pan to cool and refrigerate. Keep stored in a covered container.

Nutrition: Calories: 327 Fat: 31g Protein: 7g Carbs: 8g

Maple Custard

Preparation time: 15 minutes

Cooking time: 2 hours

Servings: 4 people

Ingredients:

- 2 egg yolks
- 2 eggs
- 1 cup heavy cream
- 1/2 cup whole milk
- 1/4 cup brown sugar
- 1 tsp maple extract
- 1/4 tsp salt
- 1/2 tsp cinnamon

Directions:

1. Combine all the fixings into a stand mixer and blend on medium-high. Oiled six 4-ounce capacity

ramekins, then put the batter into each, filling each only 3/4 way.

2. Put 4 ramekins on the bottom of the slow cooker. Arrange the other 2 on top of the bottom ramekins.
3. Cook within 2 hours on high. Remove from the slow cooker and cool to room temperature for 1 hour, then place in the fridge to chill for 2 hours. Enjoy with some sugar-free whipped cream and a sprinkle of cinnamon!

Nutrition:

Calories: 190

Fat: 18g

Protein: 4g

Carbs: 2g

Raspberry Cream Cheese Coffee Cake

Preparation time: 15 minutes

Cooking time: 4 hours

Servings: 4 people

Ingredients:

Cake Batter:

- 1 1/4 almond flour
- 1/2 cup swerve sweetener
- 1/4 cup coconut flour
- 1/4 cup protein powder
- 1 1/2 tsp baking powder
- 1/4 tsp salt
- 3 large eggs
- 6 tbsp butter melted
- 2/3 cup water
- 1/2 tsp vanilla extract

Filling:

- 8 oz. cream cheese
- 1/3 cup powdered Swerve Sweetener
- 1 large egg
- 2 tbsp whipping cream
- 1 1/2 cup fresh raspberries

Directions:

1. Oiled a 6-quart slow cooker.
2. For the cake batter, mix the almond flour, sweetener, coconut flour, protein powder, baking powder, plus salt in a medium bowl. Mix in the eggs, melted butter, plus water, then set aside.
3. For the filling, beat the cream cheese plus sweetener until smooth. Mix in the egg, whipping cream, plus vanilla extract.
4. Put about 2/3 of the batter in the prepared slow cooker. Put the cream cheese batter over the batter in the pan and spread evenly. Put the raspberries.

5. Put the rest of the batter over the filling in a small spoonful. Bake on low within 3 to 4 hours. Allow cooling completely before serving. Serve and enjoy!

Nutrition:

Calories: 239

Fat: 19.2g

Protein: 7.5g

Carbs: 7g

Pumpkin Pie Bars

Preparation time: 15 minutes

Cooking time: 3 hours

Servings: 16 bars

Ingredients:

Crust:

- 3/4 cup shredded coconut, unsweetened
- 1/4 cup cocoa powder, unsweetened
- 1/2 cup raw sunflower seeds, unsalted or sunflower seed flour
- 1/4 teaspoon salt
- 1/4 cup sweetener
- 4 tablespoons butter softened

Filling:

- 1 29 oz. can make pumpkin puree
- 1 cup heavy cream
- 6 eggs

- 1/2 teaspoon salt
- 1 tablespoon vanilla extract
- 1 tablespoon pumpkin pie spice
- 1 teaspoon cinnamon liquid stevia
- 1 teaspoon pure stevia extract
- Optional: 1/2 cup sugar-free chocolate chips

Directions:

1. Process all the fixings for the crust in a food processor. Oiled bottom of a slow cooker.
2. Press the crust batter onto the bottom of the slow cooker as evenly as possible. Put the filling fixings to a stand mixer and blend.
3. Mix in or top filling using the optional chocolate chips if desired. Pour batter onto the crust. Cover and cook on low within 3 hours.
4. Uncover, then let it cool 30 minutes, then refrigerate for at least 3 hours. Slice and serve!

Nutrition: Calories: 151 Fat: 12.4g Protein: 5.4g Carbs: 6.2g

Lemon Custard

Preparation time: 15 minutes

Cooking time: 3 hours

Servings: 4 people

Ingredients:

- 5 large egg yolks
- 1/4 cup freshly squeezed lemon juice
- 1 tbsp lemon zest
- 1 tsp vanilla extract
- 1/2 tsp liquid stevia
- 2 cups whipping cream or coconut cream
- lightly sweetened whipped cream or whipped coconut

Directions:

1. Mix the egg yolks, lemon juice, lemon zest, vanilla, and liquid stevia in a medium bowl. Mix in the heavy

cream and divide the batter among 4 small ramekins or jars.

2. Put a rack in the bottom of the slow cooker, then put the ramekins on the rack. Put enough water to reach half of the ramekins. Cover and cook on low within 3 hours.

3. Remove, then let cool at room temperature, then chill thoroughly in the refrigerator (about 3 hours). Top with whipped cream and serve.

Nutrition:

Calories: 319

Fat: 30g

Protein: 7g

Carbs: 3g

Apple Brown

Preparation time: 10 minutes

Cooking time: 4 hours

Servings: 4 people

Ingredients:

- 3 lbs. cooking apples, cored and in 2-inch pieces
- 10 slices of bread, broken into small pieces
- ¾ cup brown sugar
- ¼ teaspoon nutmeg, ground
- ½ teaspoon cinnamon, ground
- ½ cup butter, melted
- 1/8 teaspoon salt

Directions:

1. Put the apples in the slow cooker. In a bowl, assemble and mix bread cubes and all other ingredients and spread them on top of the apples. Cook within 2 ½ to 4 hours on low.

Nutrition:

Calories: 142

Carbs: 29g

Fat: 2g

Protein: 1g

Baked Custard

Preparation time: 15 minutes

Cooking time: 3 hours

Servings: 4 people

Ingredients:

- 3 eggs, beaten lightly
- 1/3 cup sugar, granulated
- 1 teaspoon vanilla
- ¼ teaspoon ground nutmeg
- 2 cups of milk

Directions:

1. Assemble and mix milk, eggs, vanilla, and sugar in a bowl. Grease a small baking dish, pour the mixture, and drizzle some nutmeg.

2. Add 1 ½ or 2 cups of water to the baking dish, cover it in an aluminum foil, and place on a rack in the slow cooker—Cook for 2 ½ 3 hours on high. Serve.

Nutrition:

Calories: 102

Carbs: 14g

Fat: 3g

Protein: 0g

Caramel Rum Fondue

Preparation time: 15 minutes

Cooking time: 2 hours

Servings: 4 people

Ingredients:

- 1 bag (14 oz.) oz. caramels
- 2/3 cup whipping cream
- ½ cup miniature marshmallows
- 2 to 3 teaspoons rum

Directions:

1. Assemble and cook the whipping cream and caramels in a slow cooker. Cook within 1 hour and 30 minutes on low and make sure the caramels have melted. Add and mix the rum and marshmallows and cook for 30 minutes longer. Serve.

Nutrition: Calories: 125 Carbs: 25g Fat: 2g Protein: 1g

Triple Chocolate Mess

Preparation time: 10 minutes

Cooking time: 6 hours

Servings: 4 people

Ingredients:

- 20 oz. chocolate cake mix
- 6 oz. chocolate chips
- 4 eggs
- 4 oz. instant chocolate pudding mix
- 1 cup of water
- 1-pint sour cream
- ¾ cup oil

Directions:

1. Grease the slow cooker. Assemble all ingredients and coon for 5-6 hours on low. It comes out better if you do not lift the lid while cooking. Best served with ice cream.

Nutrition:

Calories: 190

Carbs: 21g

Fat: 11g

Protein: 2g

Rice Pudding

Preparation time: 10 minutes

Cooking time: 5 hours

Servings: 4 people

Ingredients:

- ¾ cup short-grain rice
- 15 oz. evaporated milk
- 2 cups of water
- 1/3 cup white sugar
- ½ cup raisins
- 1 ½ teaspoons vanilla
- ¾ teaspoon salt
- 3-inch cinnamons stick

Directions:

1. Assemble all the ingredients and stir well in a slow cooker. Cook on low for 2 to 2 ½ hours on high. Stir a few times in between. Serve.

Nutrition:

Calories: 232

Carbs: 52g

Fat: 2g

Protein: 4g

Caramel Pie

Preparation time: 10 minutes

Cooking time: 7 hours

Servings: 4 people

Ingredients:

- 15 oz. sweetened milk, condensed
- 1 9-inch graham cracker crust
- 8 oz. frozen whipped topping, thawed
- 1 ½ oz. English toffee-flavored candy bars, coarsely ground

Directions:

1. Cook condensed milk in a slow cooker for 6-7 hours, whisking every 30 minutes. Pour into the cracker crust and let cool.

2. Sprinkle the whipped topping and on top of that, sprinkle the ground candy bar. Cover and refrigerate. Serve.

Nutrition:

Calories: 125

Carbs: 25g

Fat: 2g

Protein: 1g

Berry Cobbler

Preparation time: 15 minutes

Cooking time: 2 hours & 30 minutes

Servings: 4 people

Ingredients:

- 1 ¼ cups all-purpose flour
- 2 tablespoons sugar
- 1 cup of sugar
- 1 teaspoon baking powder
- ¼ teaspoon cinnamon, ground
- 1 egg, lightly beaten
- ¼ cup non-fat milk
- 2 tablespoons canola oil
- 1/8 teaspoon salt
- 2 cups raspberries, unsweetened
- 2 cups blueberries, unsweetened
- 2 cups reduced-fat vanilla frozen yogurt

Directions:

1. Assemble 1 cup flour, baking powder, 2 tablespoon sugar, and cinnamon in a bowl. Assemble the egg, oil, milk, and mix both the bowls' contents to make them into a batter.
2. Grease a slow cooker and spread the batter evenly. In a bowl, assemble the salt, the rest of the flour, and sugar. Toss in the berries and coat them—Cook for 2 and 30 minutes on low. Serve.

Nutrition:

Calories: 153

Carbs: 25g

Fat: 5g

Protein: 1g

Minty Hot Fudge Sundae Cake

Preparation time: 15 minutes

Cooking time: 4 hours & 30 minutes

Servings: 4 people

Ingredients:

- 5 tablespoons baking cocoa
- 1 cup packed brown sugar
- 1 cup all-purpose flour
- 2 teaspoons baking powder
- 1/8 teaspoon almond extract
- ½ teaspoon vanilla extract
- 2 tablespoons melted butter
- ½ cup evaporated milk
- 5 oz. mint Andes candies
- 1 cup boiling water
- ½ teaspoon salt
- 4 teaspoons instant coffee granules

- Whipped cream, vanilla ice cream, and maraschino cherries

Directions:

1. Assemble the flour, brown sugar, 3 tablespoons cocoa, salt, and baking powder in a bowl. In another bowl, assemble the extracts, butter, and milk.
2. Mix the contents of the two bowls and place them in a greased slow cooker. Crush and drizzle the candies on top.
3. Assemble the coffee, water, and the rest of the brown sugar and cocoa. Pour this mixture over the slow cooker. Remember not to stir.
4. Cook for 4 hours and 30 minutes on high. Serve with whipped cream, vanilla ice cream, and maraschino cherries.

Nutrition: Calories: 280 Carbs: 0g Fat: 13g Protein: 5g

www.ingramcontent.com/pod-product-compliance
Lightning Source LLC
Chambersburg PA
CBHW071111030426
42336CB00013BA/2033